What Others Are Saying . . .

"A beautiful devotional for those of us that know the struggle of weight and eating deeply. Marlene walks us through day by day to receive the fullness of the grace of God. I love her fun and faith filled prayers to help even with dark chocolate! This devotional is a must read and is also a big loving hug."
Jendayi Harris
Author of The Chubby Church Books
http://www.thechubbychurch.com

"*Grace and Weight* might be about the thousandth book I've read on shedding rebellious pounds that refuse to leave my body . . . but this book uniquely comforts and encourages me. Marlene honestly and cheerfully shares her battles with scales, numbers, and chocolate delights. *Grace and Weight* begins and ends with the love of Jesus for all of us who carry love/hate relationships with food and even ourselves. Here we find practical help, freedom from shame, and wonderful hope."
Lynne Babbitt, MA
Psychotherapist

"The Christian devotional book *Grace and Weight* by Marlene Bagnull is a jewel. Marlene is entirely transparent about her life-long struggles with losing weight. She provides grace and hope to help others on their weight loss journey."
Susan U. Neal, RN, MBA, MHS
Best-selling author
7 Steps to Get Off Sugar and Carbohydrates

In *Grace and Weight,* Marlene Bagnull paints an accurate word picture of the trials of losing weight and learning to eat in a healthy manner as unto the Lord.

She openly and honestly discusses the discouragement, the self-disgust, and the temp-tations we face as we subconsciously eat to fill emotional needs that only God can fill. But Marlene reminds us that no matter how powerful these habits may be and no matter how weak we might have become, God's love, His promises, and His grace are stronger. God's understanding is without limit, and His mercy is new every morning.

As you read this book, you'll be encouraged to love yourself more fully, to pray and obey instead of *wishing* for change, and to trust God more completely through the process.

Barbara Haley
Author

"I love this little book! It's a gem that has it all: humor, true confessions, road-tested tips, Scripture, and prayers. If you struggle to navigate issues related to weight or grace, this book will leave you lighter in spirit as well as pounds! I was encouraged by Marlene's transparency and wisdom, and uplifted by how each day's Scripture spoke to the challenges I face. Perfect for gift-giving, solo reading, or reading with friends, this book delivers inspiration and grace for the journey. Any book dealing with weight can be a tricky item to give to someone, right? But Marlene's writing is so authentic, heartwarming, and encouraging that anyone who receives it will consider it a blessing." **Karen Linamen Bouchard**
Author
Just Hand Over the Chocolate and No One Will Get Hurt

Grace and Weight

Encouragement for Dieters

Marlene Bagnull

Ampelos Press

Grace and Weight: Encouragement for Dieters

© 2020 by Marlene Bagnull

ISBN: 978-0-9821653-4-8

Published by Ampelos Press, 951 Anders Road, Lansdale, PA 19446
https://writehisanswer.com/Ampelospressbooks, mbagnull@aol.com

Editor: Barbara Haley
Front cover photo: Lukas from Pexels
Back cover: Image by kalhh from Pixabay
Inside art: www.Pixabay.com

Printed in the United States of America

To those who struggle
with excess pounds,
Jesus loves you!

Contents

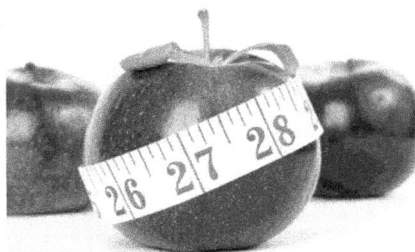

Let's Get Started

Give your bodies to God. Let them be a living sacrifice,
holy—the kind he can accept.
When you think of what he has done for you,
is this too much to ask?
Romans 12:1

Thirty-seven years ago, I made a commitment to write this book and lose 33 pounds. Sadly, I never got much further than an outline. I did lose a few pounds, but I put them back on.

Several years ago, I did lose 70 pounds. Although I still had more to lose, it felt so good to fit in clothes I thought I'd never be able to get back into. (I could open a clothing store with all the clothes I have in various sizes that I've hung onto hoping to one day wear them again.) I vowed to never gain back the pounds I lost. Of course, I did! Well, not all of them. I'm still 43 pounds less than my highest weight. But since this still puts me 72 pounds overweight (more than that according to the charts of "ideal" weight), I'm not happy with myself.

And then I wonder about God. How does He feel about my excess pounds? Do they cause Him to love me less?

Grace—One definition in *Webster's* is "divine favor unmerited by humankind." Mark Yaconelli in *The Gift of Hard Things* says, "Ultimately, grace can never be earned. Like all gifts it can only be received, requiring that I simply open my hands and trust."

I am encouraged by the words of Scripture. "He has showered down upon [me] the richness of his grace—for how well he understands [me] and knows what is best for [me] at all times" (Ephesians 1:8). My heavenly Father knows how hard it is for me to eat what I should and not eat what I shouldn't.

To echo the apostle Paul's words: "I don't understand myself at all, for I really want to do [to eat] what is right, but I can't. I do [I eat] what I don't want to—what I hate" (Romans 7:15). But it tastes so good! Still I praise God "there is now no condemnation awaiting those who belong to Christ Jesus" (Romans 8:1).

Yes, I need to lose weight, and this time I need to keep it off—for good. That will not cause God to love me more, but it will please Him because He wants me to be healthy and strong. I have His promise and so do you. "Now [we] have every grace and blessing; every spiritual gift and power for doing his will are [ours]" (1 Corinthians 1:7).

So, let's get started, not on yet another diet but on a new way of thinking and eating.

Father, please make this a joy-filled journey!

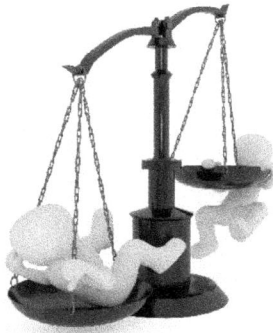

For more encouragement and prayer support, join me in the Grace and Weight Facebook group.

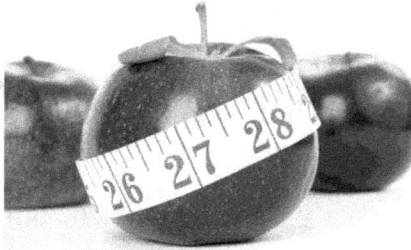

Day 1

But I Don't Eat that Much!

God has given us an appetite for food
and stomachs to digest it.
But that doesn't mean we should eat more than we need.
1 Corinthians 6:13

I've always resisted counting calories, and I detest kitchen scales almost as much as the bathroom scale. Unlike the scale in my bathroom I can "adjust" by the way I lean, kitchen scales can't be fooled.

Perhaps I can blame my childhood or at least use it as an excuse.

Because my father was a diabetic, my mother tried to follow the diet his doctor had prescribed. She carefully measured and weighed everything she gave him to eat, only to endure his complaints that she was starving him. (I didn't have a happy or stress-free childhood!)

You can imagine my dismay when I was diagnosed with Type 2 diabetes about 40 years ago. At least I don't need to give myself shots of insulin every morning as I watched my father do. But I do stick myself with a tiny needle most mornings to check my blood sugar. (I know I should check it throughout the day, but I don't like needles either.)

I would be a challenge for a weight loss coach, but since I can't afford one, I need to get over my hang-ups.

While I consider both the kitchen and bathroom scale to be a "necessary evil," they are tools I need to use. But as for counting calories, I have found a solution.

I'm an enthusiastic believer in a resource I found online. MyFitnessPal.com* does for me what I don't have the time or patience to do for myself. Its database provides the calorie count for most everything I eat. I still need to measure or weigh some foods unless that information is already on the package label. (Yes, I do read labels. It's a carryover from all the cereal boxes I read as a child.)

MyFitnessPal.com does more than just give me the number of calories in the food I'm about to consume. It also tracks the nutrients—things like fats, carbs, and proteins. Since I hate math, I love that it does all the calculations and so much more.

---

* There is no charge for MyFitnessPal's basic program. I am not paid for this recommendation.

By faithfully recording everything I eat, it's clear there is a reason for the pounds I gain. I do eat more than I realize!

As I endeavor each day to eat what I need—not more than I need or what I crave rather than what is good for me—I'm grateful for what Jesus said. "Remember, your Father knows exactly what you need even before you ask him!" (Matthew 6:8).

So, let's be certain to ask Him if what we plan to eat is okay with Him. (He does tell us in Philippians 4:6 that we are to "pray about everything.") And let's weigh and measure our food rather than tell ourselves "I don't eat that much!"

Thank You, Father, for giving me so many good and healthy food choices. Forgive me when I choose to overeat. Help me, please, to control my appetite.

BE HONEST

A kitchen scale is
as important as
a bathroom scale!

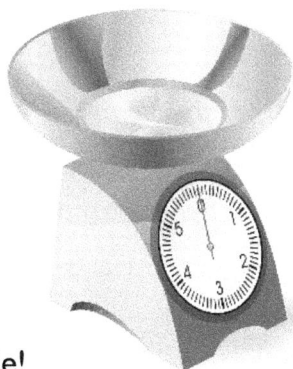

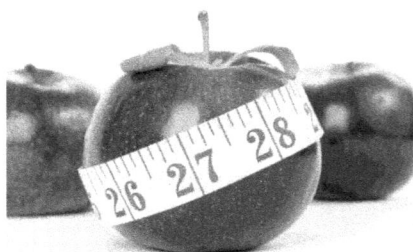

Day 2

Overcoming Temptation

No temptation is irresistible.
You can trust God to keep the temptation
from becoming so strong
that you can't stand up against it,
for he has promised this and will do what he says.
1 Corinthians 10:13

I want just one little bite, I told myself.

Okay, I lied! I wanted more than just one little bite of the extra chewy dark chocolate brownie.

The truth is one bite leads to another bite and then another.

I want and need to lose weight. The pain I've been experiencing in my knees has made it obvious that I either lose weight or face the replacement of not one but both of my knees. So, this time I've made a serious commitment to do it.

Just one bite of the extra chewy dark chocolate brownie that is calling my name isn't an option because I know I lack the willpower to stop with just one bite.

How can I, can you, overcome the temptation to believe the lie that convinces us to take that dangerous first bite?

I've begun posting Scriptures on the refrigerator and above the kitchen counter where I'm sure to find goodies. (Just because I'm trying to diet doesn't mean I can deprive my husband of food he enjoys.) Better still, I'm working at digesting (memorizing) Scripture promises.

"No temptation is irresistible," I remind myself. "[I] can trust God to keep the temptation from becoming so strong that [I] can't stand up against it, for he has promised this and will do what he says" (1 Corinthians 10:13).

But God won't remove the temptation. It's up to me to use some common sense and not leave food on my "do not eat" list where I can see it every time I walk into the kitchen.

I know "God is at work within [me], helping [me] want to obey him, and then helping [me] do what he wants" (Philippians 2:13).

Does this mean extra chewy dark chocolate brownies must forever be on my "forbidden list"? Perhaps. Or I can be wise and cut the pan of brownies into truly bite-size pieces, wrap them individually in foil, and put them in the freezer where they will hopefully remain out of sight and out of mind.

It works with the Dove dark chocolate peanut butter pieces that came in the mail from CVS. Between the scrunched box and summer heat, they melted into odd shapes. Even now that they are refrigerated, it's difficult to unwrap them. That gives me time to reconsider eating more than one. It helps that patience is not one of my virtues!

Father, please help me to put my mind on things far more important than chocolate, even dark chocolate that is supposed to be healthier. Forgive me when I get so self-absorbed in my wants and desires. I want to obey You and live—and eat—the way You want me to.

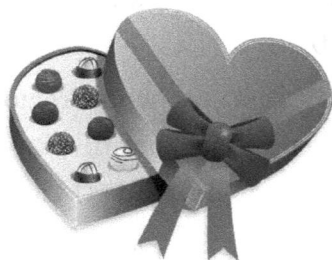

EXERCISE COMMON SENSE

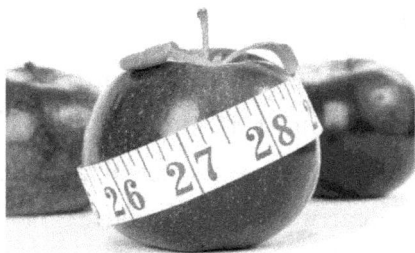

Day 3

Think on These Things

Fix your thoughts on what is true and good and right.
Think about things that are pure and lovely,
and dwell on the fine, good things in others.
Think about all you can praise God for and be glad about.
Philippians 4:8

It's no wonder I overeat. How can I resist when I spend so much time thinking about food?

Yes, I need to plan what I'm going to have for meals and check out the calorie count and nutrients in MyFitnessPal.com. That's important and needed. But letting my mind wander to the carton of chocolate peanut butter ice cream in my freezer isn't wise or good. (I do crave chocolate!)

Father brought the above Scripture to mind. It does give me a lot to think about besides food.

Thinking about what is good for me, I know losing weight and keeping it off is definitely not just a good thing but also the right thing for me to do. The extra pounds I'm carrying not only are hard on my knees, they sap my energy. Doctors say 10 pounds are equal to 40 pounds of pressure on my knees. Try carrying a 10-pound sack of potatoes just for a couple of minutes. It's certainly not something we would want to carry around day after day. And I'm not carrying just one 10-pound sack of potatoes but almost four. No wonder I'm exhausted much of the time!

What is pure and lovely? I planted strawberries this year. Seeing more bunnies than usual, I was careful to put netting around the strawberry patch. The plants were growing like the weeds I'm so good at cultivating. I thought about the luscious red strawberries I hoped to soon pick.

One morning I was horrified to see the plants had been chewed to the ground. *How did bunnies manage to get through the netting?* I wondered. Then I heard and saw a dove trying to get out of the patch. I pulled back the netting, but the dove chose to escape through the chain link fence. Yikes! If a dove could fit through, so could the bunnies. I had no idea.

Much as pictures of pie a la mode and two-layer chocolate cake covered with dark chocolate icing make my mouth water, is anything as pure and lovely as a bright red strawberry sparkling in the morning dew or the shiny purple eggplant I'm ready to harvest?

As for thinking about the fine, good things in others, that does not mean I should covet the metabolism of those who can eat, as my mother would have said, "until the cows come in," but not gain a pound. Instead I need to focus on all the reasons I have to be thankful. I don't daily face starvation as much of the world does.* I can and do praise God that not only do I have enough to eat, but I have had a wonderful variety of food available even during the scarcity of toilet paper that the pandemic created.

Thank You, Father, for all You have provided for me. Help me to think on these things and on how You are calling me to serve You and others today.

---

* "The United Nations World Food Program (WFP) has warned that by the end of the year (2020), more than 260 million people will face starvation—**double** last year's figures." https://www.cbsnews.com/news/hunger-crisis-coronavirus-pandemic/

FOCUS

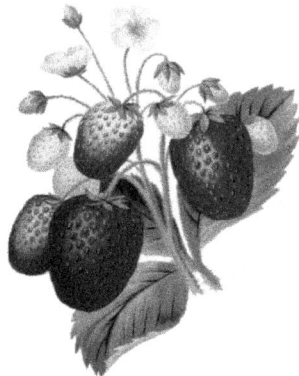

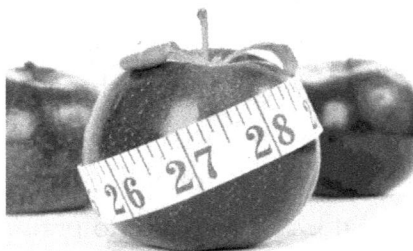

Day 4

Truth or Consequences

*So if you're serious about living
this new resurrection life with Christ,
act like it.*
Colossians 3:1 MSG

"If every day were like today, you'd weigh _____ pounds in 5 weeks," MyFitnessPal.com tells me after I finish logging in what I've eaten all day and the exercise I've hopefully done.

If I am sticking to my plan, it's great motivation to keep on keeping on. If I have consumed too many calories and have not exercised, it's a wake-up call that I'm not going to like what I weigh in 5 weeks.

I'm reminded of the old *Truth or Consequences* TV show. (Yes, I'm old enough to remember it.) The choices I make throughout the day will determine what message I'll see on MyFitnessPal.com. Its computers will calculate the truth and reveal the consequences—good or bad. If I intentionally record fewer calories than I eat (in other words, if I cheat), it will look like I'm going to weigh less in 5 weeks. But I'll be disappointed, for the consequences will be based on the truth of what I've actually eaten, not on a lie or wishful thinking.

I can depend on the fact that God doesn't lie, and I can trust in His promises. But when I carefully read the Scriptures, more often than not, I discover there is a condition attached to His promises. He has given me the freedom to choose how I will respond.

To paraphrase Colossians 3:1, "So if I'm serious about losing weight, I need to act like it."

Father, forgive me when I treat losing weight like a game. It's time I stop yo-yo dieting. Help me, please.

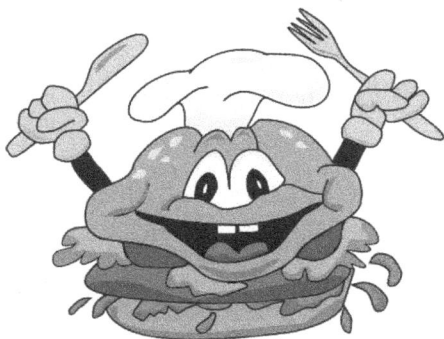

GET SERIOUS!

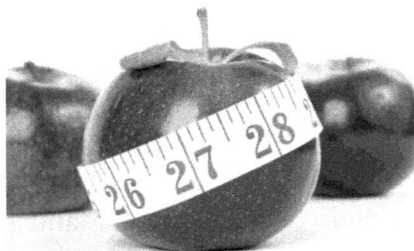

Day 5

Dieting Is Hard Work

It is quite true that the way to live a godly life
is not an easy matter. But the answer lies in Christ.
1 Timothy 3:16

Dieting is big business! As sure as the sun will rise and set each day, new weight loss plans and pills will regularly be introduced. It's tempting to believe the before and after testimonies and pictures. I know. I've fallen for a few over the years. But the fact remains, "Dieting is hard work."

One word I've learned to look out for is "miraculous." Seriously? Stop and think. If there was a miracle diet or pill, the word would spread like wildfire. No one would be overweight—well no one, that is, who could afford to purchase it. That's another red light. If it's ridiculously expensive, I've learned it's best to be skeptical. Instead of believing the hype, it's wise (and safest) to check it out with my doctor. But let's be honest with ourselves. It is tempting to look for and take the easy way out of whatever challenge we're facing.

I remember my struggle with math when I was in elementary school. Night after night I'd sit at the dining room table sobbing. "It's too hard. I can't do it!" High school algebra was even worse. It just didn't make any sense. Today I still struggle with math. I'm grateful for calculators and that I never had to contend with the "new math" my grandkids are learning.

Back to my lifetime struggle with my weight, looking through old picture albums, the only time I was thin was when I was seven or eight. Other pictures remind me of the times I was called "fatty" and other mean names. My mother was wrong when she said, "Sticks and stones may break my bones, but names will never hurt me." And I've never forgotten how embarrassed and ashamed I felt when, as an already insecure high school freshman, a teacher pulled me aside to lecture me about my weight.

Then there was the friend I had back in high school who could eat a whole carton of ice cream (and the cartons were bigger sixty years ago) and yet not put on a pound. Although she complained her butt was too big, she never weighed more than 110 pounds.

I don't know why I have been "blessed" with the propensity to gain weight just looking at food. It doesn't seem fair. And I admit I'd love for God to make it easy for me to stick to a diet and lose weight.

The first time I ever felt God speaking to my spirit He said, "Child, I never said it would be easy to follow Me, but I have promised always to be with you."

I wonder, would I need Him as much if things, including dieting, came easy? Probably not.

Father, I'm sorry for the way I grumble and whine about my struggle to lose weight. Help me to learn the lessons You want to teach me.

QUIT WHINING!

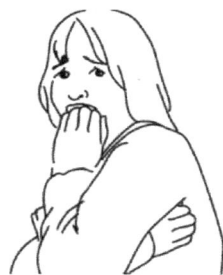

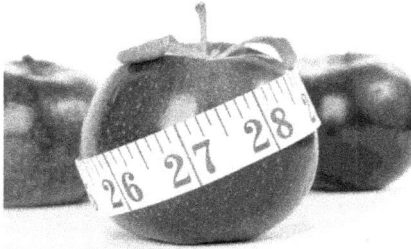

Day 6

Stress Eating

Let him have all your worries and cares,
for he is always thinking about you
and watching everything that concerns you.
1 Peter 5:7

Someone has said a picture is worth a thousand words. Drawing isn't a gift I possess, so you'll need to picture this in your mind: A wild-eyed woman is clutching a big bag of potato chips in one hand and stuffing a fistful in her mouth with her other hand. The caption reads: "I'm not stressed!"

Stress may not cause us to look wild-eyed, but it is likely to cause us to consume food without thinking. We can call it "just nibbling," but let's face it, we're likely to nibble more than we realize. We're horrified when we finally have the courage to get on the scale, but we deserve those pounds we've put on.

Now picture one of those graphs that have become so familiar during the pandemic. This one represents the weight gained each week from a cross-section of women who tend to be overweight. I have no doubt the curve would be trending up and not flattening.

The past months of lockdowns, mask-wearing, and social distancing have been stressful. For some it's been a life-altering time with the loss of employment. And tragically, for others the pandemic has caused the loss of loved ones.

We hope and pray that a vaccine will soon be available that will put an end to the coronavirus, but invariably we'll encounter another crisis. None of us are immune. Jesus sought to prepare His disciples, and to prepare us, for hard times. He said, "Here on earth you will have many trials and sorrows; but cheer up, for I have overcome the world" (John 16:33).

Christians are not promised that life will be easy, but Jesus has promised, "I am leaving you with a gift—peace of mind and heart! And the peace I give isn't fragile like the peace the world gives. So don't be troubled or afraid" (John 14:27). I don't think it's stretching the truth of this Scripture to add, "And don't use food to try and ease your stress."

What does Jesus want us to do when we're confronted with a stressful situation? And let's be realistic. More often than not, it won't be just one situation that is causing us to stress. What can we, should we, do? Instead of reaching for comfort food, let's reach for Him. After all, "He knows what it is like when we suffer and are tempted, and he is wonderfully able to help us" (Hebrews 2:18).

Thank You for Your promises, Lord. When life overwhelms me, help me to turn to You and to Your Word rather than to reach for unhealthy snacks.

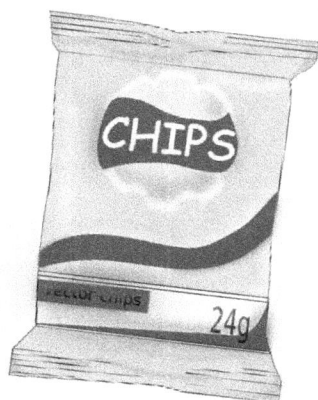

REACH FOR JESUS, NOT SNACKS!

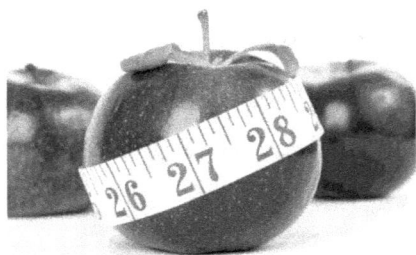

Day 7

Little Things Do Matter

"Learn to be wise," he said,
"and develop good judgment and common sense!"
Proverbs 4:5

Tonight, we had BLTs with the first tomatoes of the season from my garden. One wasn't quite ripe, but I couldn't resist picking it. I fried the bacon until it was nice and crisp to reduce its calories. (No limp, half-cooked bacon for me. I gag on it.) Toasting two slices of low-calorie bread, I was well on the way to a delicious, nutritious, and low-calorie dinner.

If only I had thought to check the label on the jar of mayo before I spread a generous amount on my toast. I should have known better, but mayo is something I don't often use. But really—what was I thinking? Of course, there were calories in the mayo, but 180 calories! Time to add low-calorie mayo to the shopping list if I'm going to have more BLTs this summer.

Until tonight I had done well sticking to my diet. What a disappointment to have blown it with just two tablespoons of mayo! Seemed like such a small amount— such a little thing. I surely was not exercising wisdom or common sense.

It's the little things that so often trip me up, and I'm not thinking just about food. Far too often I'm prone to turn a little problem into a B I G issue. My mother used to call it, "making a mountain out of a molehill." Or I'll find an hour has passed when I intended to spend only a little time on social media.

Then there are those times when I compare where we're at financially with others our age and indulge in self-pity. Or I'll complain that I have so little time to do things I'd like to do. And there's the biggie of the little things that I allow to take priority over giving the Lord first place in my life and living as He wants me to (see Matthew 6:33).

Father, please forgive me when I let little things derail me. Remind me to come to You not just with big things but with little things as well.

SEEK
WISDOM

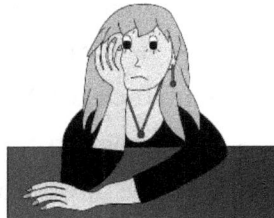

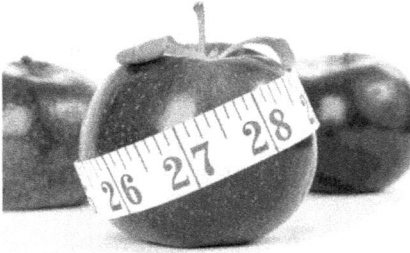

Day 8

Workouts

Workouts in the gymnasium are useful,
but a disciplined life in God is far more so,
making you fit both today and forever.
1 Timothy 4:8 MSG

There must have been a flock of birds outside our window early this morning. Their chirping woke us from a sound sleep. "What on earth," I groaned as I crawled out of bed to look out the window.

Then it hit me. It was the alarm on my iPhone! I had set it the night before, so I'd wake up in time to reserve one of the lap lanes at the pool. There are only six time slots available for each 45-minute swim. It's becoming more popular since the YMCA reopened a month ago, and now it's a challenge to reserve the time I prefer since it can only be done the day before.

I've been swimming Monday through Friday for the past 24 days, and I don't want to break my record. At half a mile each day, I've swam 12 miles in the past 5 weeks!

You won't find me in the Y's gym on a treadmill or elliptical. If that works for you, great, but it doesn't work for me. Years ago, I purchased an exercise bike. After the first week, it became a handy place to pile clothes.

The important thing for all of us chubbies is to find an exercise that we'll stick with over the long haul and that will burn up those calories. It needs to be a real workout, not a leisurely stroll through Walmart's candy aisle. And if we have health issues, it needs to be doctor approved.

Keeping fit is important, and not just keeping physically fit. Even more important is keeping spiritually fit through making prayer and the study of God's Word a daily priority. "Every part of Scripture is God-breathed and useful one way or another—showing us truth, exposing our rebellion, correcting our mistakes, training us to live God's way" (2 Timothy 3:15 MSG).

Father, I know these things. Please help me to do them!

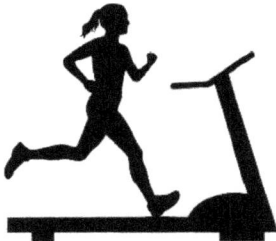

KEEP FIT

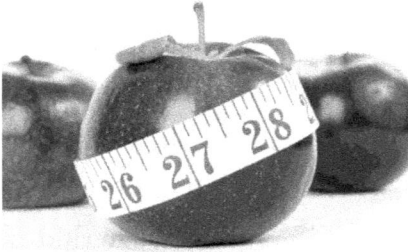

Day 9

Look Before You Leap

*I can do everything God asks me to
with the help of Christ who gives me the strength and power.*
Philippians 4:13

I grew up watching *The Adventures of Superman* on our black and white, small screen television. Mild-mannered Clark Kent amazed me when he transformed into the guy with the big "S" on his chest who could leap tall buildings in a single bound. Perhaps I have him to thank for my "I'm invincible and can do anything" attitude.

That attitude has often gotten me in over my head when without thinking, much less praying, I've said yes to things God was not asking (or equipping) me to do. It's no wonder I frequently feel overwhelmed because there are not enough hours in the day to accomplish all I have foolishly over committed myself to do.

Yes, it's time I learn to look before I leap!

The other day I stopped at Chick-fil-A on the way home from swimming. My husband likes to eat dinner before 6:30, and I hadn't been able to reserve an earlier lane at the pool. So, I had a good excuse to get dinner at Chick-fil-A. The calories (without the bun) were reasonable, and I shared the waffle fries with Paul.

But I saw something I wish I hadn't seen. A new Freddy's Steakhouse Restaurant was behind Chick-fil-A. I'm a hamburger gal. Since the next evening I also had the later swim time, I stopped and got a patty melt. It didn't sound like it contained a lot of calories. It was on rye bread instead of a bun and looked (and was) luscious.

Unfortunately, I also saw Freddy's has onion rings. Of course, I ordered them along with French fries. I again shared the fries with Paul, but I was happy he only wanted one onion ring. But . . . I was not happy later when I looked up the calories on MyFitnessPal.

Unbelievable! The patty melt was a whopping 760 calories, the French fries (I ate more than half) were at least 300 calories, and the onion rings (good grief) weighed in at 600 calories. Not only did I eat up the 643 calories I burned swimming, with Freddy's grand total of 1,660 calories I was 460 over the calories I am trying to stick to every day. And that didn't include the calories I consumed eating breakfast and lunch.

Will I never learn to listen to the still, small voice of the Holy Spirit?

Oh Father, please help me to listen for Your voice when I am tempted, rather than to leap and eat. And help me to stay away from fast-food restaurants.

COUNT THOSE CALORIES!

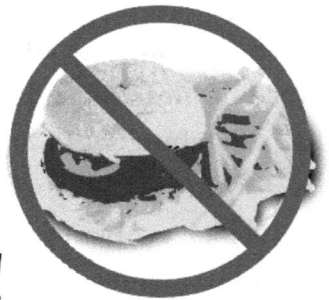

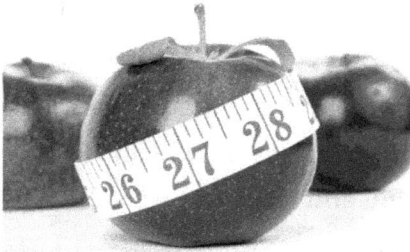

Day 10

Reminders from Above

*And we know that all that happens to us
is working for our good
if we love God and are fitting into his plans.*
Romans 8:28

There has not been one hummingbird at my feeder or anywhere in my garden this spring or summer. But this morning, I spotted one perched in a tree above where I was watering the lawn. Suddenly, it started flitting in and out of the spray of water.

I had been having one of those "terrible, horrible, no good, very bad days" that started yesterday afternoon when the keyboard on my laptop stopped working. Almost two hours on the phone with technical support exhausted my patience and, sadly, provided no solutions. "You'll need to reformat your hard drive and reinstall Windows," the tech said.

No way, no how! There are just too many programs and files on my laptop. Reformatting is way beyond my expertise or patience.

I called Windows support. I was put on hold and listened to their elevator music for over two and a half hours. I finally gave up waiting and went to bed.

This morning, I overslept, probably subconsciously trying to avoid the inevitable. At least the backup I ran last night using a virtual keyboard worked, but I forgot to back up the ton of important emails I have organized in folders. Because I direct two large writers' conferences there are just too many to print. Besides, I think it's important to save trees! Backing up is not a quick or easy process, and I admit I foolishly take chances and rarely run a backup. While the computer hummed away, I decided to water my thirsty garden. I hadn't gotten it done last night because I was waiting for tech support.

As I continued to grumble, the hummingbird appeared. I thanked Father for sending one of His creatures to lighten my foul mood.

What does this story have to do with "grace and weight"?

When I'm frustrated (and nothing can make me more frustrated than my computer), I typically reach for food.

But thank the Lord I chose to take care of my plants that were crying for water instead of stuffing food in my mouth. It helped that it was still morning. Somehow, I've managed to train myself not to snack in the a.m. If only I could master that skill for the rest of the day!

God's grace was also evident when this time, after I finished watering, I was able to reach a Windows tech. Amazingly, he resolved the problem in five minutes. God did work all things together for good since my laptop is now backed up. It was L O N G overdue and a risk I should not have been taking.

Father, on those days when nothing seems to be going right thank You for the reminders that are all around me that You are able to work all things for good. You are the answer—not food!

LEARN TO LAUGH

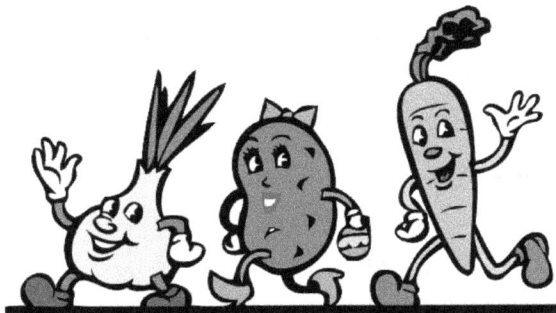

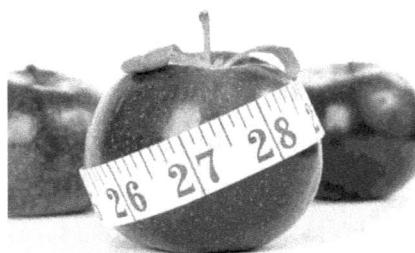

Day 11

Patiently Waiting

*Patience develops strength of character in us
and helps us trust God more each time we use it
until finally our hope and faith are strong and steady.*
Romans 5:4

I've always found it hard to wait for things. As a youngster, it seemed like forever from one special day to the next. I'd count the days until Christmas and Easter, the end of the school year, and my birthday.

When someone thought I was older than I really was, I'd grin from ear to ear. (That has definitely changed!) I was thrilled when I passed the test for my driver's license, but I was frustrated that I had to wait until I had a job and enough money to buy a car and pay for my own insurance.

After Paul and I were married in 1963, I continued to find it difficult to wait. Nine months of being pregnant with our first child stretched three weeks past my due date. It didn't seem fair that I was also late with our two other babies.

I didn't have the patience to wait until we could afford things our growing family needed, so we ended up deep in debt. I learned that failing to patiently wait for things can have serious consequences.

The maturity that comes from lessons learned the hard way has made me a little more patient, but I've still got a long way to go.

One thing that continues to try my patience is the scale. I'm working hard at getting the pounds off. I'm swimming five days a week and pretty much staying within the calorie count that should make me weigh less when I step on the scale. And I am losing, but two pounds in ten days seems so S L O W.

Just as my children used to whine about how long it was taking to get somewhere just minutes after I backed out of the driveway, I whine about how long it's taking to lose weight.

There are days when I'm tempted to give up. But "Finishing is better than starting! Patience is better than pride!" (Ecclesiastes 7:8). I need to "keep on patiently doing God's will [I know He wants me to lose weight] if [I] want him to do for [me] all that he has promised" (Hebrews 10:36).

Father, forgive my impatience. Help me to keep on keeping on, trusting You to help me reach my weight loss goal.

KEEP ON

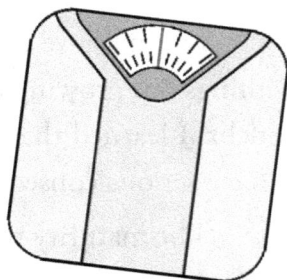

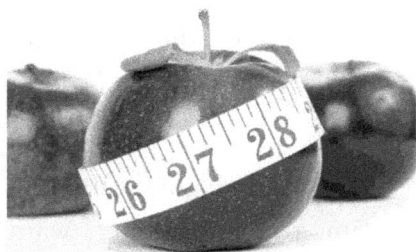

Day 12

Don't Give Up!

Wait passionately for GOD, don't leave the path.
Psalm 37:34 MSG

Yesterday I complained (yes, I really was complaining) about how long it takes to lose even a couple pounds. Duh! Of course, it takes time. My weight loss goal, actually *any* goal, will only be reached if I stick to it. In other words, I need to make up my mind not to give up no matter how long it takes.

One of my daughters used to ice skate competitively. Part of her training included practicing school figures. Not only did it take time and patience to master the intricate figures, it must have been boring. I found it much more exciting to watch her free skate. The jumps and spins she attempted often took my breath away—especially when I saw her fall. But Debbie got up again and again. She kept trying and didn't give up.

43

Debbie has always been passionate about succeeding at whatever she does. Good thing. Otherwise she never would have gotten through all the years it took to become a pediatrician. Book learning was hard, but those all-night rotations during her internship were grueling. I don't know that I could have done it.

I can't count the number of times I've gone on a diet only to give up. I so want this time to be different. I want and need to succeed. But how, when I've failed so many times in the past?

Fact is, I can't succeed in my own strength. Instead of complaining about my "thorn" of being overweight, what if I embrace it? I didn't say accept it. Instead, what if I thank God for the struggle I have to control my weight and allow Him to use my weakness to draw me closer to Him?

Father, I want to experience the blessing the apostle Paul discovered as he battled his "thorn." Through my struggle, show me how "When I am weak, then I am strong—the less I have [including will power], the more I depend on [you]" (2 Corinthians 12:10).

PERSIST

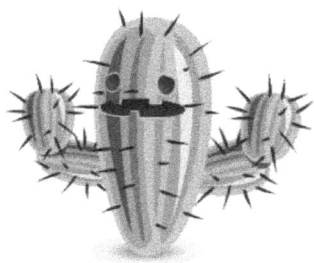

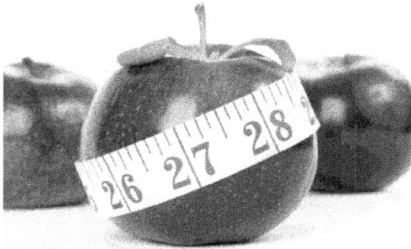

Day 13

Willpower or God Power?

But when the Holy Spirit controls our lives
he will produce this kind of fruit in us:
love, joy, peace, patience, kindness, goodness, faithfulness,
gentleness and self-control.
Galatians 5:22-23

"I can't do it," my daughter wailed. "You do it for me, Mommy."

Every morning I heard the same thing. And every morning I showed her—again—how to tie her shoelaces. My patience was wearing thin. "You're not trying," I said. "Come on. I know you can do it if you try."

I never succeeded in teaching her how to master this skill. Gratefully, a teacher in nursery school did.

Fifty years later I often hear myself echoing my daughter's words. In fact, to be honest, almost every day (and sometimes throughout the day) I tell the Lord, "I can't." Usually it's a computer glitch I can't figure out or the deadlines of directing two conferences that can cause me to feel totally overwhelmed.

Sometimes God sends someone to help me. Other times He waits for me to calm down so that I can hear His voice. But I never sense Him becoming impatient or annoyed with me. He doesn't accuse me of not trying hard enough.

"God helps those who help themselves," is a familiar saying. Some think it's in the Bible, but it's not. Erwin Lutzer says, "More often God helps those who cannot help themselves, which is what grace is about."

Yes, I need to use the intelligence God gave me. And when it comes to sticking to my diet, I need to exercise willpower. But did you know another word for willpower is self-control? And it's a fruit of His Spirit.

Thank You, Father, for reminding me of that old hymn, "I Need Thee Every Hour." I do! I'm so grateful that the willpower I need is God power and it's a fruit of Your Spirit working within me.

BEAR FRUIT

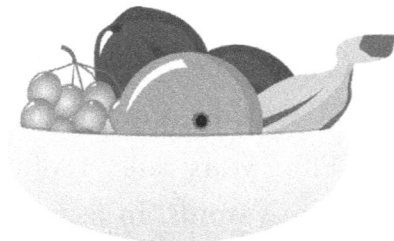

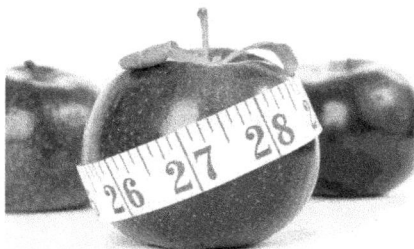

Day 14

Discouraged

Why am I discouraged? Why is my heart so sad?
I will put my hope in God! I will praise him again—
my Savior and my God!
Psalm 42:11 NLT

I overdid it today, and my knees are screaming in protest.

The morning was cool, and thanks to the eight to ten inches of rain from Tropical Storm Isaias, I knew I would be able to get my spade through our hard clay soil to dig up some perennials I'd been wanting to move to another part of the yard.

I headed to Lowes to get some topsoil. I should have asked someone to load the bags in my car, but I hate being a helpless old lady. Besides, there were only three bags. But then I needed to unload them when I got home. I heaved two of them into our wheelbarrow. Another mistake. I should have loaded just *one* bag in the wheelbarrow, so it wasn't so heavy to move. But that would have meant making two trips across the uneven ground in our backyard.

By now it wasn't as cool, and the sun had moved into the garden that had an abundance of daylilies and hostas that I needed to divide.

Of course, I got overheated. I did have enough sense to take a (short) break and gulp down a glass of water. But then, even though I was exhausted, I knew I needed to get what I had dug up replanted. At least now I was able to work in semi-shade. Good thing since the mercury was climbing.

Time flew as it always does when I work in my garden, and before long it was time to head to the pool for my daily 45-minute swim. Swimming half a mile was especially hard today, but I pushed myself and did it.

After dinner I had to retrieve my kneeling pads from the garden since it was supposed to rain. I could hardly pull myself up the two steps onto my porch.

Growing old isn't for wimps! And trying to do what I've always been able to do isn't easy with two bad knees. It makes losing weight not an option. If only I'd remember that when I'm tempted to eat food that comes with a guarantee that it will put on pounds.

Father, please transform my discouragement into renewed determination to persevere in this battle to lose weight.

STAY DETERMINED

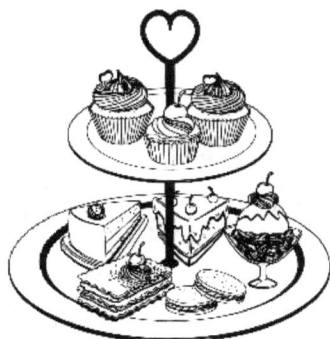

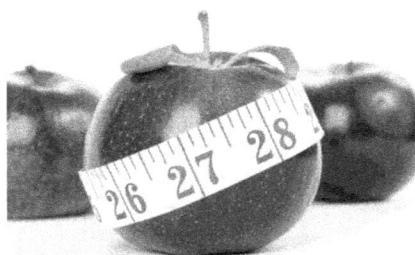

Day 15

Are You Motivated?

Keep your eyes open, hold tight to your convictions,
give it all you've got, be resolute.
1 Corinthians 16:13 MSG

"Your son is smart, but he doesn't apply himself," I heard at every parent/teacher conference. "He could be at the top of his class if he only tried, but he's just not motivated."

All through elementary and middle school we kept hearing the same thing from Robbie's teachers as he continued to get mediocre grades. When he entered high school, the "you can be anything you want to be" speech didn't motivate him, nor did the threat that he was limiting his college options and the possibility of receiving much needed scholarship help.

We were amazed when Rob was accepted by his first-choice college and even more amazed when he received a small scholarship. Within a month of graduating from college he landed a job in his career field. Clearly it was God's grace.

I've also experienced God's grace. He has protected me from the serious health problems that are associated with obesity. (I hate that word!) But I doubt He is going to miraculously heal my arthritic knees that are now bone on bone. The only way I'm going to avoid the replacement of both knees is to lose weight. Surely that should be the motivation I need.

What about you? The desire to look good is probably not going to be enough to motivate you to persevere. But those sacks of potatoes you are carrying that sap your energy and can medically have serious consequences can be the needed wake-up call.

Father, forgive me for how I have allowed myself to become obese. I want and need to take better care of me.

WAKE UP!

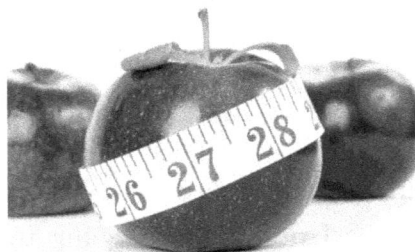

Day 16

The Gift of Encouragement

So speak encouraging words to one another.
Build up hope so you'll all be together in this,
no one left out, no one left behind.
1 Thessalonians 5:11 MSG

Today was my 30th day at the YMCA pool. The lady who checks me in made the motion of balloons dropping from the ceiling. We high-fived through the plexiglass barrier to prevent the spread of the coronavirus. She has been cheering me on each day she is on duty. She has even told me more than once that she is proud of me!

Words of encouragement are such a precious gift. Knowing how much they mean to me, I look for opportunities to encourage others.

When was the last time you encouraged yourself? I felt the Lord ask me.

I was stunned by His question. Although I'm known as an encourager, it has not occurred to me to speak encouraging words to myself. Instead, most days I'm likely to do the opposite. I focus on the things I do wrong (or my efforts that are not good enough) rather than acknowledge and cheer myself on for the good things I accomplish.

"Quit beating up my friend," someone said to me a number of years ago.

I had forgotten her admonition.

What about you? When was the last time you gave yourself a well-deserved pat on the back? Do you celebrate the days you stick to your diet—and not by rewarding yourself with a bowl of ice cream?

Lord, You know how easy it is for me to put myself down. No wonder I become discouraged. Help me to guard my thoughts.

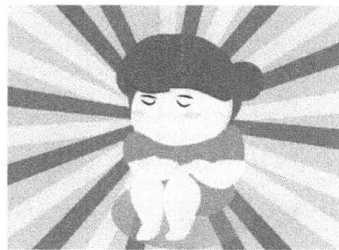

GUARD
YOUR
THOUGHTS

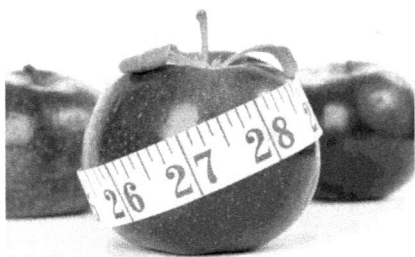

Day 17

Put Downs

"And you will know the truth,
and the truth will set you free."
John 8:32

The years I spent in elementary school were some of the most unhappy years of my life. Everyone in my class had a special friend—everyone but me.

There was an uneven number of kids in my class. Maybe that's why I never had a partner when we had to line up in pairs. But why me? Why didn't anyone want to walk with me? And why was I always the last one to be picked for a team in gym class? I couldn't help it that I was a klutz. What was even worse were the "Oh crap, we got stuck with Cripe (my maiden name) from Mars" comments from my classmates. I would have given anything to change my first and last name.

Sadly, they were not the only mean words I endured. I was ridiculed for the clothes I wore and laughed at when my tongue got twisted on "ch" and "sh" words. Being pulled out of class for speech therapy only added to my embarrassment and heartache.

Things weren't any better during summer vacation. The schoolyard was right across the street from my house. My father insisted I live out his dreams and play baseball. He had been a star pitcher in high school and was scouted by the Chicago White Sox. He got injured and became seriously ill with tuberculosis. I don't think he ever got over his disappointment I wasn't a boy.

At some point during those years I began turning to food for comfort. Now "fatso" was added to the names I was called. It was many years before I finally was able "to feel and understand, as all God's children should, how long, how wide, how deep, and how high [God's] love really is" (Ephesians 3:18). As my pastor's wife said, "Even if I was the only person on this earth, Jesus still would have come and died just for me."

Thank You, Lord, for loving me and never giving up on me.

CUT THE TAPES

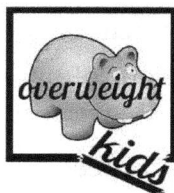 become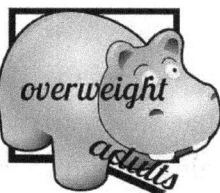

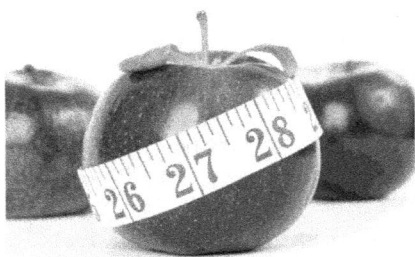

Day 18

What's for Dessert?

Search me, O God, and know my heart;
test my thoughts.
Psalm 139:23

Even though my father was a diabetic on insulin, he insisted that no dinner was complete without dessert. My mother loved to bake and to please him, although she did try to limit the amount of sugar in the recipes and to control the size of what she served him. She would often hide what was left of a pie or cake she baked.

I was raised to expect and automatically ask, "What's for dessert?" Six and a half decades later, I've suddenly realized how much that childhood expectation still influences me. And it's just one of my attitudes about food that are a carryover from my childhood. Not only has my mind been programmed to expect dessert after dinner (or a bowl of ice cream in the evening), food is a necessary part of celebrations and a comfort when I'm hurting or stressed. I need to pay attention to what Benjamin Franklin said and "eat to live, not live to eat."

Romans 12:2 tells me I need to "be transformed by the renewing of [my] mind." And that word from the Lord applies to so much more than just food.

The entire verse reads, "Do not conform to the pattern of this world, but be transformed by the renewing of your mind. Then you will be able to test and approve what God's will is—his good, pleasing and perfect will."

Just as it's all too easy to treat myself to dessert after dinner, it's also all too easy "to go along with the crowd" and not take a stand for what I know is right. Especially in today's culture wars, I need to listen to and support the voices that line up with the truth of God's Word.

Father, please reprogram my mind to think Your thoughts. I want "my spoken words and unspoken thoughts" (Psalm 19:14) to please You.

RENEW YOUR MIND

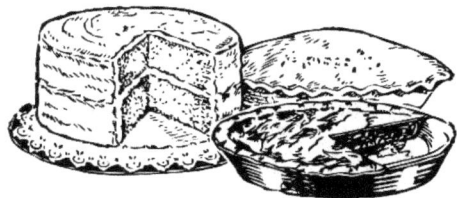

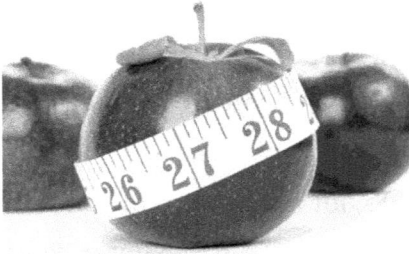

Day 19

What Do You Know?

*You must learn to know God better
and discover what he wants you to do.*
2 Peter 1:5

There's a lot I know, but there's also a lot I don't know and need to know!

Fats make me fat. Sugar is dangerous. Protein is important, but red meats are not the most healthy source. Vegetables are good for me, but some are not as good as others. Carbs are high in calories. Whole grain bread is better than white bread.

Good grief. I don't sound very knowledgeable, do I?

Fact is, I'm not! I need to make it a priority to learn more about the foods I'm eating, should not be eating, and should eat.

Proper nutrition is a complex topic. Just as someone has said, "Rome wasn't built in a day," my gaps of knowledge will not be filled overnight. But there is plenty of information available so there is no excuse to remain ignorant about something that is so important. But where do I start? And how do I guard against scams?

My mother used to say, "If it sounds too good to be true, it probably is too good to be true." Diets that promise quick weight loss through extreme measures are tempting but best avoided. Not only are they likely to deprive my body of needed nutrients, weight lost quickly also comes back on quickly.

I believe in the old (but not old-fashioned) food pyramid adjusted for my needs as a diabetic. There are lots of examples online along with the serving size of foods in each part of the pyramid. Many even include daily menus. Now I just need to find one that I can tailor to my likes and dislikes. And then comes the hard part—exercising the needed discipline to follow it faithfully.

Father, please help me to identify and to appreciate the healthy foods You have provided for me. You are a good, good Father.

CHOOSE WISELY

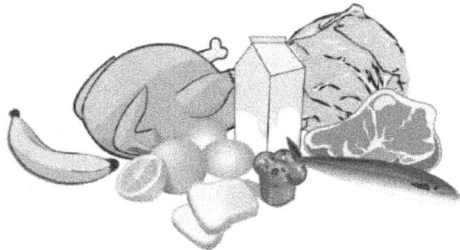

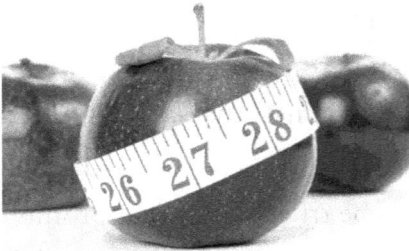

Day 20

Discipline

To learn, you must love discipline;
It is stupid to hate correction.
Proverbs 12:1 NLT

Growing up I was all too familiar with discipline. My father would routinely slap me across the face, throw me in the bedroom, and lock the door. I was terrified when he came after me. He was a huge man who weighed well over 300 pounds. Other times he would pick up the phone and ask the operator to connect him with the police so he could ask them to come and take me away since I was a "bad little girl."

One definition of discipline, according to *Merriam-Webster*, is "punishment by one in authority especially with a view to correction or training." But I never understood what I had done to make my father so angry or what he was trying to teach me. He rarely talked to me except to yell at me. I don't remember ever sitting on his lap. He never told me that he loved me.

I am so grateful for how God has healed my childhood memories. I now know that He is my heavenly Father, that He loves me, and that I do not need to fear His discipline. "It's the child [God] loves that he disciplines; the child he embraces, he also corrects" (Hebrews 12:6 MSG).

Just as God uses discipline to show that He loves me, I need to love myself enough to exercise wise self-discipline. When I mess up (and I do and I will), I can choose to learn from my mistakes rather than beat myself up for failing. And I can rest in the fact that my Father loves me.

Father, thank You for loving me enough to keep correcting and training me to be all that You know I can be.

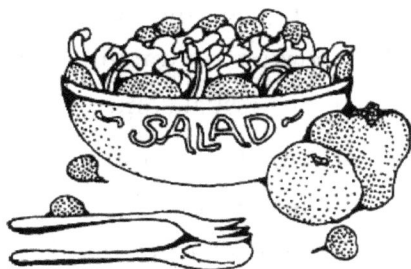

PRACTICE HEALTHY SELF-DISCIPLINE

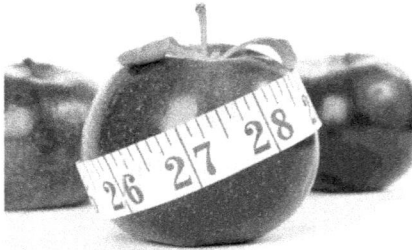

Day 21

Habits

*Let your enthusiastic idea at the start
be equalled by your realistic action now.*
2 Corinthians 8:11

I've heard and believed that it takes 21 days to make or break a habit. That's good news because it feels like something I should be able to do with God's help. So, I've been working on watching what I eat and recording it daily on MyFitnessPal.com.

Okay, I admit I've missed a day here and there. But I just read online that researchers have found that "missing one opportunity to perform the behavior did not materially affect the habit formation process."*

---

* "How Long Does it Actually Take to Form a New Habit? (Backed by Science)" at https://jamesclear.com/new-habit.

Whew! This same article went on to say, "In other words, it doesn't matter if you mess up every now and then. Building better habits is not an all-or-nothing process."

My relief was short-lived as I continued to read. Twenty-one days is not the magic number. Instead, a scientific study determined it can take anywhere from 18 to 254 days to form a new habit! A bit of good news is that the average is 66 days. But 66 days! I want to be well on my way to reaching my weight loss goal by then, not just gotten started.

Through the years I've enthusiastically started more diet plans and weight loss programs than I can count. Sadly, I've been successful only a couple of times. Even then, I've failed to keep the weight off.

"Why, God?" I asked Him this morning.

He called my attention to the word *realistic* in the above Scripture.

It's not realistic for me to expect to quickly lose the pounds I've gained. Nor is it realistic to create a new habit in 21 days, 66 days, or even longer. Fact is I have a lifetime of bad eating habits I need to change, and that's going to require a long-term commitment to creating new healthy habits.

"I don't think I can do it," I told the Lord.

"You're right, you can't in your own strength," He said. "But I will help you."

Father, please turn my discouragement into determination and realistic action.

BE
REALISTIC

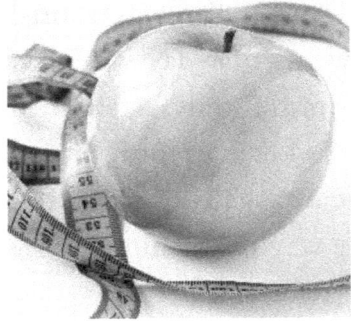

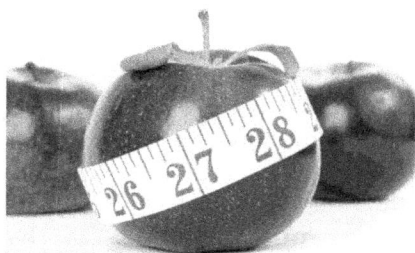

It Takes Time

*Let your roots grow down into him
and draw up nourishment from him.
See that you go on growing in the Lord, and become
strong and vigorous in the truth you were taught.*
Colossians 2:7

"Fifty pounds in 61 days!"

Lately that subject line has been popping up in my bulk email folder. I haven't bothered to open it, although it has caught my attention. It would be great if it were true, but not only is it spam, it's impossible! But I admit I did peek and read, "New No-Exercise 'Skinny Pill' Melts Belly Fat." Wow . . . but no way. I did *not* click the link!

A magic pill capable of dissolving pounds! Unbelievable, yet some desperate chubbies will, no doubt, purchase it. I wonder if it's a money-back offer if you're not satisfied? Don't worry. I'm not about to find out.

It's been exactly a month since I began writing these devotions for you and for myself. I've pretty much stuck to 1,200 to 1,500 calories a day (after the 600 or so calories I get credit for burning off swimming laps).

How much have I lost? Not much! Only 3.5 pounds— a far cry from the 25 pounds I would have lost on the "miracle" pill.

Am I discouraged? A little. I don't want it to take this much time even though I know this is a healthier way to lose weight and keep it off. But then, I always have been one who strives and drives myself to accomplish the goals I set—goals that far too often are unrealistic. I'm sure you've already discovered that I'm not a patient person. As a result, I can be my own worst enemy and sabotage my success by giving up when something takes longer than I think it should.

But with Father's help, NOT this time. If I have to go on a bread and water diet (I won't, although I do love bread with lots of butter), I'm going to stick to it.

Just as my growth as a Christian is something I've been working on since I was fourteen and asked Jesus to forgive my sins and be Lord of my life, I'm going to keep working to lose the weight I never should have allowed myself to gain. In the process, I'm trusting my life will "overflow with joy and thanksgiving for all he has done" and will do (Colossians 2:7).

Father, thank You for the true miracle of Your enabling power that is better than any magic pill.

PERSEVERE

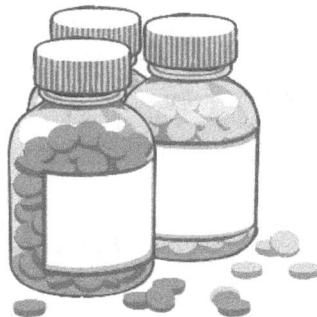

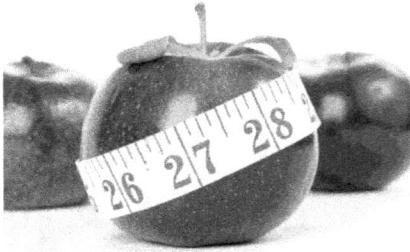

Day 23

Star Light, Star Bright

*When I pray, you answer me and encourage me
by giving me the strength I need.*
Psalm 138:3

Summer is almost over. It's certainly been different than most. No swimming at the outdoor community pool. No picnics with the need to social distance. No vacation— well that hasn't happened in years with directing a summertime conference although I had to cancel this summer's conference (it would have been the 37th) because of the pandemic.

I'm feeling nostalgic tonight remembering summer evenings when I was growing up. I remember catching lightning bugs and putting them in a jar with a lid that I had carefully punched holes into so they would survive. If

I caught enough of them and they all blinked at the same time, maybe I'd be able to read after my mother made me turn off the light next to my bed.

I remember the double dares to jump off the highest level of our front porch. No wonder I now have arthritic knees. And there was the mulberry bush that we would run around, the luscious berries I'd stuff in my mouth, and my mother's scoldings because of the stains I got on my clothes.

But most of all I remember wishing on a star. I'd memorized the nursery rhyme when I was little:

Star light, star bright,
First star I see tonight,
I wish I may, I wish I might,
Have this wish I wish tonight.
Anonymous

As an impressionable pre-adolescent watching Walt Disney's *Magic Kingdom* and listening to the haunting words in "When You Wish Upon a Star," I became a believer. I wished for new clothes instead of hand-me-downs. I wished to be transformed from an ugly duckling into a beautiful princess. I wished I'd be able to make new friends when school started in the fall. And the same as all young girls, I wished for a "prince charming."

Sadly, most of my wishes never came true. I continued to wear hand-me-downs. I only remember my mother buying me one new dress. It was for my graduation from 8th grade, and it was ugly—same as me. And I never did fit in with the kids at school.

But my life began to change when I came to know the Lord and my wishes became prayers. He gave me three special friends in high school and a relationship with Him that was more important than clothes and trying to look beautiful. And I know He introduced me to the man who I've been married to for 57 years—my "prince-charming."

What does all this have to do with grace and weight? Everything! Wishing will never make the pounds melt off. Only prayer will help me to eat right and continue to exercise. Gratefully, He loves to listen and to help!

Thank You, Lord, for answering my prayers and blessing me in ways so much better than my childhood wishes.

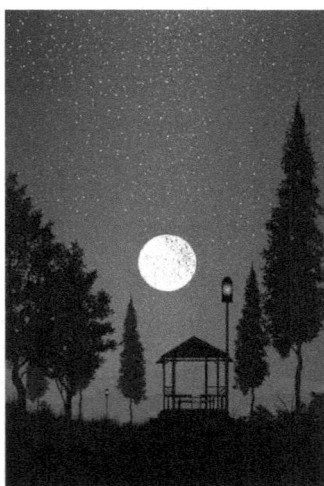

COUNT YOUR BLESSINGS

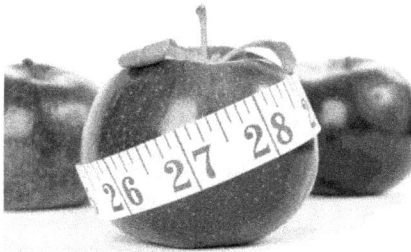

Day 24

My Favorite Things

Open my eyes to see wonderful things in your Word.
Psalm 119:18

One of my all-time favorite movies is *The Sound of Music*. I never get tired of watching scenes I know by heart. Like the night of the thunderstorm when the vonTrappe children dash into Julie Andrews' bedroom and jump onto her bed. Of course, I sing along with Julie as she tries to calm their fears by encouraging them to think about their "favorite things."

I have a long list of favorite things: hugging my grandkids—although with the pandemic it's been almost eight months, walking in the woods—although that's also a memory with my bad knees, working in my garden—I'm grateful for padded cushions and still being able to get up and down, and yes FOOD!

71

Chocolate peanut butter ice cream, Dove Chocolate Peanut Butter Silky Smooth Promises, chocolate fudge cake, brownies . . . Yes, anything chocolate! And pastries, especially my mother's icebox coffee cake I bake every Christmas.

I love homemade macaroni and cheese with, of course, tons of cheese. And how could I forget fried foods? The onion rings the staff orders at Poppy's every year after the Colorado Christian Writers Conference are the best in the world. I always order a second platter and keep it near me so I can reach for more when hopefully no one is looking.

Hmm . . . eating my favorite foods is not going to help me lose weight and thinking about them makes me want to raid the fridge.

What if I asked Father to help me revise my list of favorite foods and to give me a new appreciation (and taste buds) for what He has provided?

I suspect He would add things like strawberries (not resting on a big piece of cake and smothered with ice cream), fresh cauliflower and broccoli (minus globs of Cheez Whiz), lettuce salads (minus high-calorie dressings), lean cuts of meat (not greasy hamburgers), nutritious and filling whole grains . . .

Does that mean I can never eat my favorite foods? Of course not. I think God wants us to enjoy eating and that He delights in the creativity of chefs and bakers. But He also wants me to be healthy, which can't happen if I regularly indulge in large portions of my favorite foods.

Father, please renew my mind and transform my taste buds. Help me to learn to appreciate the simple things that are also good for me.

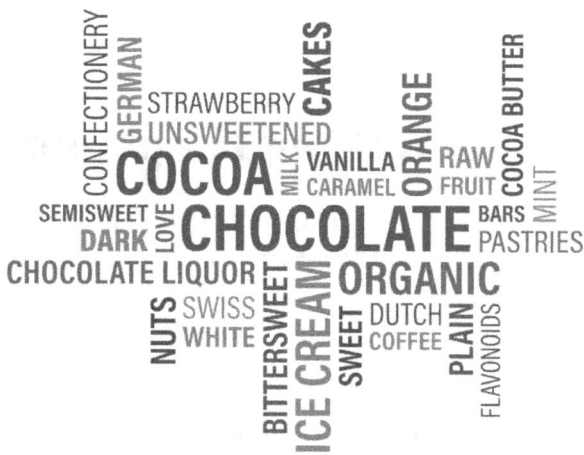

CONFECTIONERY GERMAN STRAWBERRY CAKES UNSWEETENED COCOA BUTTER ORANGE COCOA MILK VANILLA RAW CARAMEL FRUIT MINT SEMISWEET LOVE CHOCOLATE BARS DARK PASTRIES CHOCOLATE LIQUOR ORGANIC NUTS SWISS BITTERSWEET ICE CREAM SWEET DUTCH PLAIN WHITE COFFEE FLAVONOIDS

CHOOSE TO CHANGE

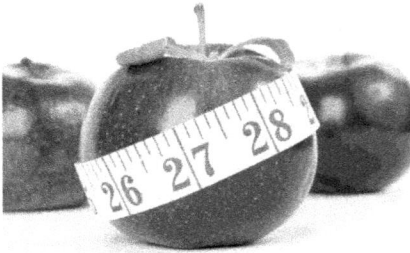

Day 25

Avoiding Temptation

"Keep alert and pray.
Otherwise temptation will overpower you."
Matthew 26:41

Turkey Hill chocolate peanut butter ice cream is on sale this week. I really, really want to add it to the grocery shopping list. I know if I do, I won't be able to limit the size of my nightly treat to just a 2/3 cup that I can have if I work those 230 calories into the number of calories I'm trying not to exceed each day.

I stayed strong and didn't add it to the list. Sigh. But I don't know what I'll do when the pandemic ends and I again am able to go grocery shopping. Right now, my daughter insists I stay home and let her get our groceries. Although I didn't add chocolate peanut butter ice cream to the list I emailed to her, I did see bakery chocolate chip cookies were also on sale. *Surely it won't hurt to treat myself to just one a day,* I told myself.

I'm sure I don't need to tell you that I didn't stop with just one cookie a day!

After all the cookies were gone, I thought again of the promise in 1 Corinthians 10:13: "No temptation is irresistible. You can trust God to keep the temptation from becoming so strong that you can't stand up against it, for he has promised this and will do what he says." But when I deceive myself into thinking I can exercise self-control (and when I fail to ask Him to help me because I really want what I shouldn't have), temptation wins.

Just as it would be foolhardy for an alcoholic to walk into a bar, I'm foolish to think I can handle the temptation of having food in the house that I know I can't resist. And it's not just that I'll be tempted to eat more than I should. Once I do, I know I'll also be tempted to believe the voice of discouragement and to give up.

Oh Father, help me not to believe the lies I tell myself. Forgive me for how I foolishly set myself up to fail.

RESIST TEMPTATION

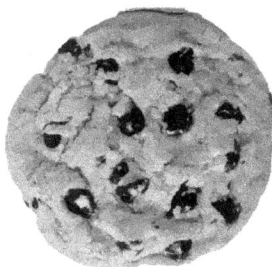

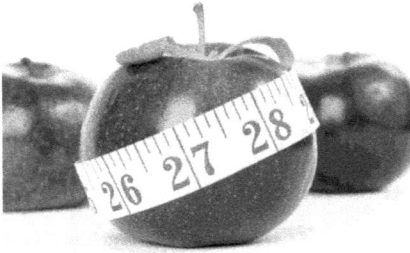

Day 26

Not This Time!

*Remember, too, that knowing what is right to do
and then not doing it is sin.*
James 4:17

The pandemic has been an excuse for many to turn to food. But truth is, if it wasn't covid-19, we could readily find or create another crisis to use as an excuse. Life is full of problems—big and small. They don't have to be crisis-size to serve as a handy excuse to use food as a comfort.

It's hard to stick to a diet and all too easy to undo the progress we've made. I know. I've been there; done that countless times. If I had a buck for every pound I've lost and gained back, I'd be wealthy!

James 4:17 convicts me: "Knowing what is right to do and then not doing it is sin." (James 4:17).

I'm not saying it is a sin to indulge in foods that are sweet and fattening—foods that are not part of a healthy diet. But it's not smart, and I'm disappointed in myself when I gain back what I've lost. The truth is, it's sinful to turn to food instead of the Lord when life gets me down. Instead, I need to

Turn [my] eyes upon Jesus,
Look full in His wonderful face,
And the things of earth will grow strangely dim,
In the light of His glory and grace.
                    Helen Howarth Lemmel (1922)

Food can never do for me or for you what Jesus wants to do. How it must grieve Him when we turn to food instead of Him. Knowing this and not doing it—not allowing Jesus to be our comfort and strength—is sin.

Forgive me, Lord, for all the times I've turned to food instead of You. Not this time, Lord. Please help me.

LOOK
TO JESUS

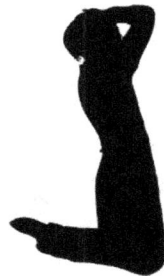

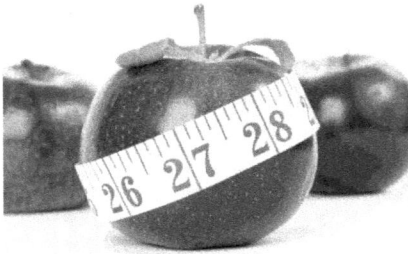

Day 27

Measuring Up

*Be a new and different person with a fresh newness
in all you do and think.*
Romans 12:2

No matter how hard I tried, I never was able to measure up to what my father expected. If I got a 98 on a test in one of my school classes, my father would yell at me for not getting 100. He always insisted I could have and should have done better and accused me of being lazy.

I kept on trying to measure up and, sadly, kept on failing. Although he died when I was only thirteen years old, the impact his words had on me never died. Even years later as an adult I found it impossible to live up to what I now expected of myself.

My defeatist attitude impacted everything I tried to accomplish. I convinced myself that I was not smart enough or good enough to achieve success. So why try? Yet I kept trying and then beating myself up when my best wasn't good enough. Yes, I did live up to my expectations. I expected to fail and so I did!

Change didn't happen overnight. It took years of not just studying God's Word but believing what I read. God loves me and has a plan for my life. He speaks words of affirmation, not condemnation. I need to speak those words to myself and rely on His promise to help me.

Of course, I still do not measure up to all I expect of myself, but now it is rare for me to turn to food for comfort. Truth is food didn't help. If anything, I used it to punish myself. After all, I'd tell myself, *I deserve to look as awful as I feel.* Wow. Talk about a negative attitude!

Learning to see myself as God sees me is a lifetime endeavor, but I praise God that each day is a new day of experiencing His loving presence and mercy.

Thank You, Lord, for the newness of life in You each day that has set me free from the spirit of condemnation.

AFFIRMED NOT CONDEMNED

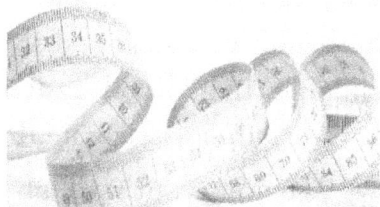

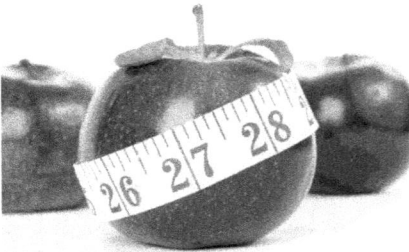

Day 28

Celebrations

Go and feast on all the good things he has given you.
Celebrate with your family.
Deuteronomy 26:11

We love to celebrate! Holidays, birthdays, graduations, weddings, anniversaries, promotions . . . no matter the reason for celebrating, one thing is certain, there will be food. Lots of food!

From October through January my family celebrates not just Thanksgiving and Christmas, but my birthday, my husband's birthday, and the birthdays of all three of our children. In addition, in January our daughter-in-law and two sons-in-law celebrate their birthdays.

Obviously, it's tough to stick to my diet during those months, especially when it comes to our traditional Thanksgiving and Christmas feast.

I don't know how anyone can resist the tantalizing aroma of roasting turkey or the table laden with family favorites on Thanksgiving. Not wanting to offend anyone, I need to at least sample every dish. And then there are the yummy desserts. My son's cheesecake rivals the Cheesecake Factory. Of course, I also need to have a slice of pumpkin pie with whipped cream.

Christmas is even harder. At least I no longer have the energy to make 12 to 15 different kinds of cookies to give away. But every gathering of family and friends provides a tempting variety of fattening and sweet treats.

Choosing to play the martyr only puts a damper on the celebration. And honestly, I don't think it's what the Lord wants me to do. He understands the role food plays in our celebrations and even established feast days for His people. But I do think He wants me to exercise wisdom. I can eat less the day or two before, and I do not need to be the one to finish the last piece of cheesecake or pumpkin pie. Someone in my family will gladly take care of that for me!

Thank You, Father, for the part food plays in our celebrations.

BE THANKFUL

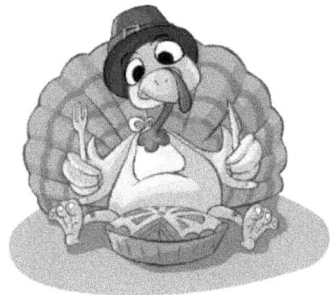

Day 29

An Egg a Day

Getting wisdom is the most important thing you can do!
And with your wisdom, develop common sense
and good judgment.
Proverbs 4:7

For years I have insisted, "An egg a day keeps the doctor away." Seriously, how can what nourishes baby chicks be anything but healthy for humans? Have I been wise to ignore the advice of experts? Not really, although I am happy to report that scientists now say the cholesterol in eggs is not as bad as once was thought.*

For many years I've also eaten a banana every day. I've never sought to justify that for health reasons. I simply love bananas. But about a year ago I discovered that bananas

_____
* https://www.livescience.com/50834-eggs-nutrition-facts.html

are not something I should be eating with chronic kidney disease. There is no controversy surrounding this information that was there all along had I made it a priority to do some research.

As I said earlier, "Proper nutrition is a complex topic." There are over 100,000 books on nutrition available on Amazon plus a ton of information that can be found on the Internet. So, there is no excuse for remaining ignorant about a topic that can seriously impact the quality and length of my life.

But where to start? On pages 91-92 you'll find books, written by Christians, that I'm in the process of devouring. Well, not literally. I still prefer eating real food! But I am grateful for the work these authors have done to equip me with the knowledge I need to make wise choices.

Father, forgive my laziness and complacency. Please help me to study and learn about the best foods to eat.

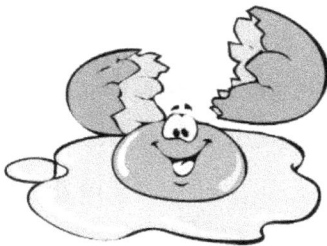

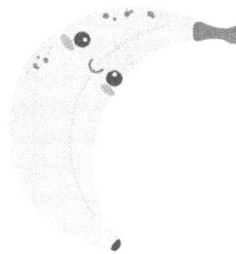

BE WISE & TEACHABLE

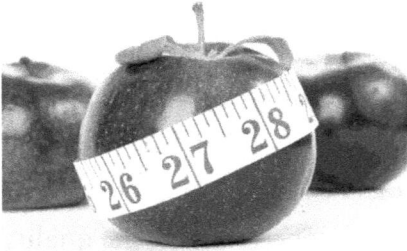

Day 30

Now to Him Who Is Able

And now to him who can keep you on your feet, standing tall in his bright presence, fresh and celebrating.
Jude 1:24 MSG

About two and a half months ago I began writing this book. I was making great progress until not one but two hard drive crashes brought my writing to a halt.

Although I was not able to record what I ate in MyFitnessPal, Father helped me not to abandon my effort to lose weight as I have too often done in the past when I'm stressed.

Nine pounds are not as much as I had hoped to lose in about ten weeks, but I could have easily *gained* nine pounds! Still it's tempting to become discouraged and to allow the excess pounds I'm still carrying to accuse me of being a big, fat failure.

I'm again drawn to the need to embrace grace in my ongoing struggle to lose weight. And I'm reminded of the song I learned as a youngster:

Jesus loves me, this I know,
for the Bible tells me so.
Little ones to Him belong;
they are weak, but he is strong.
Yes, Jesus loves me! Yes, Jesus loves me!
Yes, Jesus loves me! The Bible tells me so.
Anna Bartlett Warner (1859)

His love for me is unchanging! It is not based on whether there is more or less of me to love. Yes, I am weak, but He is strong.

To paraphrase Jude 1:24, "He can keep me from turning to food when I'm stressed. Because He is with me, I can stand in His strength." When I fail, I can embrace His grace, and rejoice in His unfailing love. So, can you!

JESUS LOVES ME AND YOU!

Laura's Prayer

My friend, Laura Shaffer, is a powerful prayer warrior. Join us in this life-changing prayer:

Lord Jesus Christ, thank You for Your grace and for Your forgiveness each time I fail. Thank You that Your love for me doesn't depend on my balance sheet of successes or failures.

Thank You for the body that You've given me. Even as far from ideal as I see myself, thank You for my strengths and for my weaknesses. Thank You that my strengths help me move forward in the motivation that You give me. And thank You that my weaknesses bring me to rely more on You.

Although I have been assured that my identity and my value come from who I am in You, and not a number on the scale or a reflection in the mirror, I want to live healthy and eat healthy to make the most of the body You've given me. Help me get real with myself and get real with You.

Heal those places in me that drive me to eat when I'm really looking for healing. Instead of eating when I feel stress, boredom, frustration, pain, or shame, let me bring those things to You.

Break my unhealthy relationship with food.

When I feel lonely, help me not be led by those feelings but remember the fact that You are with me because You have promised to never leave me.

When I feel discouraged or ashamed, help me not to be led by those feelings but to remember the fact that You love me and have accepted me as I am.

When I feel like a failure, help me not to be led by my feelings but to remember the fact that I'm only human and that I can learn through failure. Thank You that it can be a stepping-stone to success.

When I feel bored or in pain and want to eat, help me not to be led by those feelings and to try and eat them away or drown them with food. Instead, help me to trust in the fact that feelings are fleeting. They are the caboose on the train. And the engine that drives me is that I have the power to choose my actions based on the facts of Your love for me, Your purpose for me, and Your grace and forgiveness for me.

Father, You know food and eating are battles I face every day. Take away the desire I have to eat the things that are not good for me. And when I do eat what is good for me, let it be satisfying and filling.

Fill me with Your Spirit and Your purpose in a way that gives my life the meaning and satisfaction I've been looking for in food.

When I really think about it, I know that food cannot give me what I want. So, help me to quit behaving like it can. That is an infantile and childish way of thinking. Father, help me mature. Help me grow out of these childish ways of thinking to become the adult that I need to be and to live my life based on reality instead of fairy tales. Help me put aside the childish hope that someday a fairy godmother will come and wave her magic wand and transform me into a beautifully shaped princess.

The sooner I accept that there are consequences for my actions, for my eating, the sooner I can enjoy taking back control and reaping the benefits of eating what is good for me in quantities that help me achieve realistic goals.

I want to learn what is best for me, for my body, and for my health with my particular health needs, concerns, likes, and dislikes. Please teach me. Lead me to what is true, not the fad and false sensationalism in the dieting world.

Help me step forward, taking one day at a time, with Your grace and mercy renewing me every day.

This is what will bring me better health and longer life. It is what will allow my joints, heart, kidneys, pancreas, liver, and lungs to all work in the way You created them to sustain my body and allow me to do the things You created me for.

Thank You for drawing me to this book which encourages me so I can revel in the grace that You give me every day. Thank You for reminding me how much You love me and care for me. I am so grateful that You are by my side on this journey. Amen.

I encourage you to subscribe to Laura's two blogs and to purchase her encouraging booklet, *7 Ways in 7 Days to Pray THROUGH the Pandemic.*

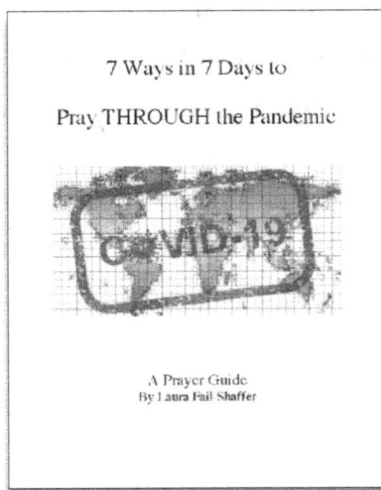

https://DailyBiblePrayer.wordpress.com

https://HearMoreFromGod.wordpress.com

Website coming soon at www.Listenup.mom

Recommended Reading

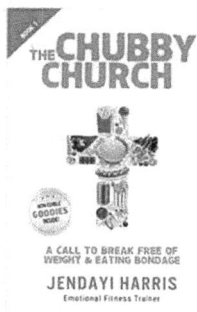

THE CHUBBY CHURCH

A CALL TO BREAK FREE OF
WEIGHT & EATING BONDAGE

JENDAYI HARRIS
Emotional Fitness Trainer

Have you tried diet after diet only to lose it and gain it back? Do you struggle with emotional eating, overeating, bread cravings, junk food, or sugar addiction? Finally, a path for victory over one of the most prevalent, yet under-discussed areas of bondage within the church: Weight & Eating Bondage.

Giving Christ First Place will guide you to discover the importance of prayer, the joy of obeying God, the truth about excuses, how you can cope with temptations, the secrets of true satisfaction and pleasing God, and how to commit yourself to do God's will.

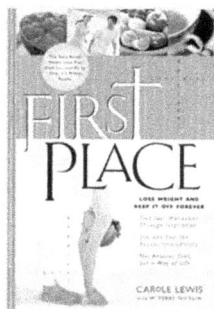

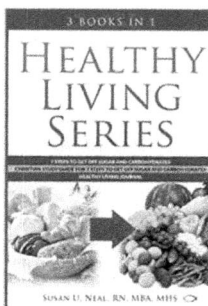

FIRST PLACE

CAROLE LEWIS

3 BOOKS IN 1

HEALTHY LIVING SERIES

SUSAN U. NEAL, RN, MBA, MHS

Determine the root causes and solutions for your ill health or excessive weight so you can experience a more abundant life and feel good again. Three books in one: *7 Steps to Get Off Sugar and Carbohydrates; Christian Study Guide for 7 Steps to Get Off Sugar and Carbohydrates; Healthy Living Journal.*

The Lost Weight Workshop will take you on a
faith-filled journey that reaches far beyond the
goal of weight loss to a place where food has
lost its hold on you. A whole new way of doing
the "diet thing" that will transform not only
your outer appearance, but your entire being:
spirit, soul and body.

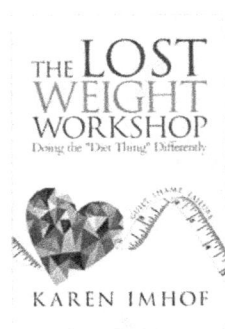

THE LOST
WEIGHT
WORKSHOP
Doing the "Diet Thing" Differently

KAREN IMHOF

All available on Amazon.

Other Books by Marlene

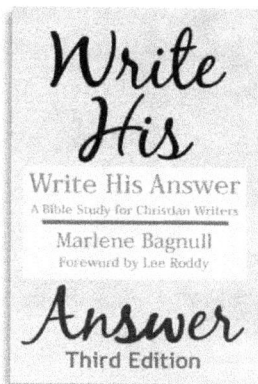

Write His
Write His Answer
A Bible Study for Christian Writers
Marlene Bagnull
Foreword by Lee Roddy
Answer
Third Edition

Now in print 28 years!
Practical help and encouragement
for overcoming self-doubts, writer's block, rejection,
procrastination, and more with Scriptures to study,
questions to apply the message to your life,
and space to write your response.
Check out the free excerpts at
https://writehisanswer.com/writehisanswerbiblestudybook

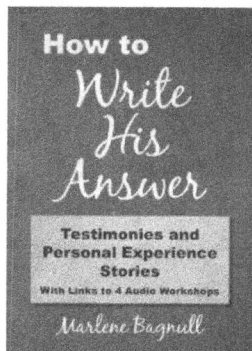

How to
Write His Answer
Testimonies and Personal Experience Stories
With Links to 4 Audio Workshops
Marlene Bagnull

Includes links to 4 audio workshops

Upcoming books in this series:
Articles & Devotionals
Fiction
Put Your Best Foot Forward
Going Indie

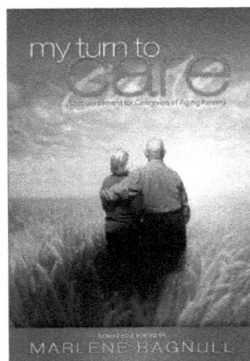

Overwhelmed by the needs of an aging parent? *My Turn to Care* will help you discover God's blessing and draw on His strength. No "how-you-can-do-it-better." Just gentle encouragement and inspiration by over 100 caregivers in the trenches.

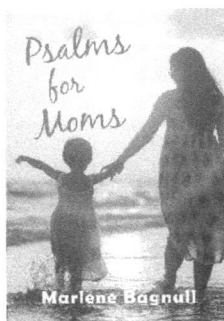

Just as the psalmist sought the Lord, I poured out my heart to Him through the daily challenges of raising three children. These psalms will encourage you to seek the Lord for everything you need to be the mother you long to be.

Childhood . . . It's supposed to be a carefree time of joyful innocence. Sadly, that is not the experience of countless children including my half-sister. Fearful she was pregnant with her father's child, Mandy came to live with us when she was not quite fourteen. *#MyFamilyToo!* is the story of God's faithfulness during the five years we sought to help Mandy overcome her father's abuse. It is also our testimony of how God helped us to Live His Answer in the midst of other challenges that could have destroyed our faith.

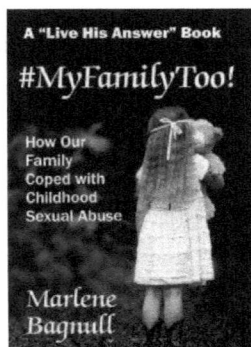

Available at www.WriteHisAnswer.com/Bookstore

Pray much for others;
plead for God's mercy upon them;
give thanks for all
he is going to do for them.

1 Timothy 2:1

**For more encouragement and prayer
visit the Grace and Weight Facebook group.**